Incorrigible optimist

9 Easy Steps with Self-Help Book to Make Your Life More Positive and Happy

Table of Contents

Introduction	3
Chapter one	
UNDERSTANDING FAILURE	14
Chapter two	
LEARN NOT TO FEAR THE FUTURE	17
Chapter three	
TRY OUT NEW, UNUSUAL AND	
DESPERATE THINGS	20
Chapter four	
BE FLEXIBLE, AMENABLE AND	
OPEN TO CHANGE	22
Chapter five	
BE POSITIVE	25
Chapter six	
PERSEVERANCE; EMPLOY HIBERNATION AND	
STANDBY MODE TO BEAT HARD TIMES	28
Chapter seven	
DO NOT GET ISOLATED; DECIDE,	
COMMUNICATE, INTERACT AND	
BE IN THE THICK OF ACTION	31
Chapter eight	
BE GRATEFUL FOR WHAT YOU HAVE	34
Chapter nine	
CREATE A BUFFER-ZONE	37
Conclusion	40

INTRODUCTION

A groundbreaking research in the Netherlands recently revealed an oft-suspected yet derided truth;

"Optimists and people who have a positive outlook on life live an average of nine more years than pessimists and people with a negative outlook and attitude".

Other similar researchers over the years have also proven an association between a higher rate of success, happiness and fulfillment, and the corresponding levels of optimism. Why then do we still seem to have more optimists than pessimists across the world? Why do most people for the seemingly safer option of expecting little or nothing from life and their prospects? Why should you seek to fill your life with hopes, expectations, and positivity?

To do that, firstly, we need to understand how our mind works, and how its pendulum swings from positivity to negativity, and ultimately, optimism to pessimism. How does it do this? First of all, our mind is divided into two voices, so to speak. One is the voice of caution, urging us to play safe, to take no risks and expect little from what we want. It is the voice that feels you not to make that investment, or start a new relationship. It is the voice that helps you imagine negative outcomes from the onset of your actions. In short, it is the center of pessimism. The other voice represents hope and ambition. It is the spark that allows you start again when you fail. It is the energy that refuels your drive and urges to succeed. This voice allows you to break new ground and attempt the undone. However, this voice has no limits or caution. It simply urges you on and gives next-to-no attention to danger or stop signs.

How then can our mind reconcile these two seemingly opposite parts and unite them into a single functioning mind? One represents an ever-depressed throttle or accelerator while the other is a permanently engaged brake that does not allow you shift even an inch except when you want to go in reverse. So, the brain establishes a balance and equilibrium between both, to give us a functioning mind. Now, the point of equilibrium differs from individual to individual. Very successful and happy people have learned to tilt their balance towards more and more optimism and rarely give their mind the chance to dwell on negativity and pessimism. They continuously seek to see the opportunities in every situation, and that is how they continue to enjoy more success and happiness. On the other hand, a chronic pessimist allows her balance to favor pessimism and the playing-safe game. She takes only the safe choices and never really gets to enjoy life to the fullest.

Have you identified yourself as a chronic pessimist? Are circumstances threatening to turn you into an incurable pessimist? Do you constantly choose the safest options to minimize the risks of being disappointed or failing? Are you simply trying to understand the benefits and difference between optimism and pessimism? Or maybe you are seeking for ways to increase your optimism and develop the right habits that can help you cement an optimistic approach to life generally? If you have answered "yes" to any of the questions above, then you are certainly in the right place right now and holding the right book.

I have purposely written this book to help you unlock the keys to optimism in your mind. I have written this book to help you tilt the scale in favor of optimism and positivity, and ultimately more satisfaction and happiness. I hope that this book can serve as a guide and tutorial for you to learn what it takes to be optimistic and how you can become an optimist. Nine proven steps and habits cannot only help you develop control over the voices in your head but keep you in control. They are;

1. Learn not to fear the future
2. Try out new, unusual and desperate things
3. Be flexible, amenable and open to change
4. Be positive
5. Perseverance; employ hibernation and standby mode to beat hard times
6. Do not get isolated; decide, communicate, interact and be in the thick of the action.
7. Give out care; identify and support somebody weaker than you
8. Be grateful for what you have
9. Create a buffer-zone

These nine steps will arm you against pessimism in all its various guises and forms. They will give you the ability to pick out the silver lining regardless of how deep or threatening the clouds seem to be. However, it is not enough to open a book on the right page. You need to read that particular page and others after it. You need to put the nine steps into action to see their effects in your daily life. Do not just read and keep aside. Act on them, act now!!!

WHAT IS OPTIMISM?

A pessimist sees the difficulty in every opportunity; an optimist sees the opportunity in every difficulty."
Winston Churchill

I may choose to give you yet another dictionary meaning of optimism, but I guess you must have had your fill of that already. So, instead, I invite you to see the true meaning of optimism by way of an illustration. Let's recount the story of J.K Rowlings, the famous author of the Harry Potter series.

In 1992, Rowlings had just lost her mother to a fatal illness she had battled for a decade. Distraught and in need of a change of scene, she decided to move to Portugal. Within the space of the next eighteen months after she had left for Portugal, Rowlings got married, had a daughter and got separated from her husband. Once again, she had to pick herself up and decided to return home to England. She had to depend on the government welfare to feed her young daughter and herself. All this while, Rowlings continued to work on the manuscripts of a seven-series book she had begun shortly before going to Portugal. Despite her present circumstances and bleak prospects, she refused to be weighed down and continued writing while holding a variety of low-paying jobs to make ends meet.

When she finished her work which she had great hopes on, she began to seek out a publisher to get her work out to the readers. Was she lucky to convince the first publisher, or the second, or the third, or the fifth? No!!! All the major publishers rejected her book citing the fact that children's books did not hold much commercial appeal. Did this kill off the hopes of this young woman? Of course not!!! She kept trying and eventually, the twelfth publisher she spoke to agree to give her book a try. However, his belief was so strong that the book would fail that he advised her to get a day job. He nonetheless published and the rest, as they say, is history. J.K Rowlings became the most popular female author of all time, became richer than the Queen of England overnight and a beacon of success and fulfillment worldwide.

J. K. Rowlings may be a household name today, but what would have happened if she had allowed pessimism stop her from completing her project? What would have happened if the initial rejections had destroyed her optimism? Well, she would have ended up like the thousands of writers better than her who have written books better than hers, but lacked the currency of optimism to see their dreams and goals come to fruition. Is hers a story of dogged determination, perseverance, and raw talent? You bet it was. However, what fuelled her determination? What gave her the energy to persevere when all seemed lost?

What allowed her to believe in her talent and refuse to give up her dream and hopes? It was optimism!!! Her beliefs that tomorrow would be better kept her awake and trying to achieve success. It made it impossible for her to give up and quit trying. Quitting was never an option because she made herself believe that success was hers, only for the trying.

This is a true definition of optimism. Optimism is to remain positively upbeat, committed and determined in the belief that future prospects would be better than what current circumstances suggest. It is to continue trying instead of believing that all is lost and quit. Optimism is that voice in your head urging you on, telling you can produce great results from your current actions and circumstances. Pessimism, on the other hand, is allowing the weeds of negativity to cripple the flowers of progress and success, under the false assumption that the odds suggest that you would fail.

An optimist cleans her mind of all negative intuition and baseless thoughts that seek to hamper her progress. She doesn't refrain from trying just because her guts tell her she would fail. Rather, she tries (and maybe fails) and then tries and tries until she can no longer fail. Optimism is therefore not just a single action or thought; it is an entire personality type and general outlook on life.

WHY YOU SHOULD BE AN OPTIMIST

"Only those who attempt the absurd can achieve the impossible."
— Albert Einstein

Optimism is not just another word coined by some distant, long-forgotten and obscure lexicographer to explain yet another psychological trait. It is in fact, a real determinant of how far you can progress and how much happiness you can derive. The thing most people fail to understand about happiness and success is that you can achieve as much of them as you permit yourself. There are absolutely no limits on the level of happiness you can extract from your life; it all depends on you and your mind.

Let me be honest; we were all born safely. Like every other animal, by default, human beings are wired to seek safety first. This is why most people who rather have no hopes than have their hopes dashed. It can sound more comforting to remain within a supposed mental comfort zone where your expectations are as low as possible, but this is actually misleading. For instance, let's examine the mind of a chronic pessimist. When a pessimist meets a new friend or prospective partner, she isn't thinking; "how may I help this relationship", "I hope this turns out great" and "he seems very nice" kind of thoughts. No, she is already on the "Is this not going to turn out like my last relationship", "why should I waste my time on another useless and futile relationship" and "this may likely be a waste of time" wavelength. As a result, she has armed her mind against the relationship even before it starts. Therefore, no matter how hard the new friend or partner and she may try, they are already fighting a losing battle.

Being a pessimist robs you of the vantage point. It has you fighting a losing battle with the word "go". By thinking of failure, you already have started to fail. Your destiny is the product of the various outcomes you experience. Your outcomes, however, are manifestations of your actions, and your actions are spurred and determined by your thoughts. Think of failure and failure becomes your most probable outcome. Think of success and you are already on the path to success. Our mind does not have a mind of its own. It takes whatever grain we put in it and produces its chaff.

What do Winfrey Oprah, Beyonce, Rev Martin Luther King, Barack Obama and Thomas Edison have in common apart from huge personal success? What is the difference between them and you? In eight letters, it is O P T I M I S M. These personalities have all surmounted unbelievable odds to leave a mark on the sands of time. They have all achieved their tall goals because they dared to believe. They deleted the pessimism gene in their DNA and though and acted towards success until it was no longer a possible outcome, but in fact, the only outcome left.

Optimism gives you one last chance just when you have absolutely exhausted all your chances. It gives you a reason to continue to keep putting one foot in front of the other even when you are totally exhausted. It keeps you going and clears a new path just when you think you are at a dead end. With optimism, no situation is too hard, no problem is too difficult, and no goal is too high. Optimism brings everything down to your reach.

This is what you stand to gain by being optimistic. We are the products of what we think and by thinking positive, you prepare your mind and change the odds to favor you in your bid to succeed and be happy.

CHAPTER ONE

UNDERSTANDING FAILURE

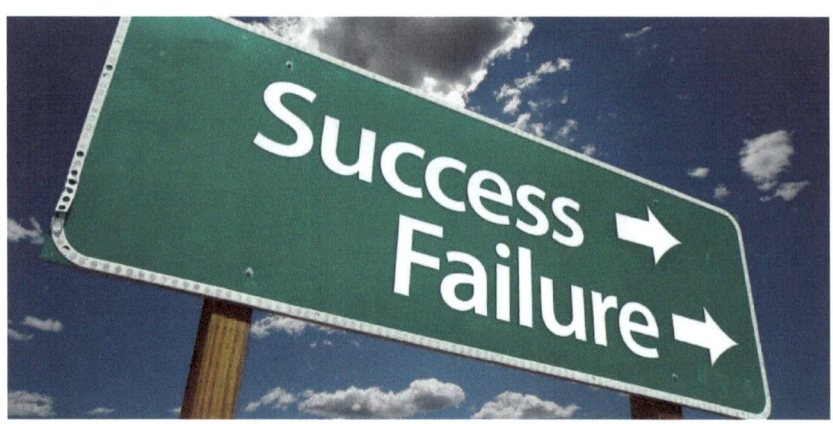

Even the darkest night will end, and the sun will rise." — Victor Hugo

The main difference between an optimist and a pessimist is their definition of failure. If you must become an optimist, you must learn to see failure from a new angle. The pessimist sees failure as a roadblock, a message to turn around and go away. Therefore, ideally, she is scared of failure. She does not want to fail at all. Therefore, she steels his mind against failure and is so cautious that she refuses to allow her success and happiness grows big.

If you must be an optimist, however, then, you need a new definition of failure. Failure is not a charge to stop; it is, in fact, a message to try harder. It is, in fact, a gate for keeping out unserious and unwilling people. Knock harder, and failure will turn to success. At worst, you may need to change your approach and try again from a different direction. Failure isn't a permanent roadblock, just a small bump along the path of success.

Thomas Edison was reported to have carried out over 10,000 experiments to perfect the light bulb. 10,000!!! What kept him going? How was he able to keep up his willpower and mental strength? Simply because, he believed he could do it. He was optimistic his skills could produce the perfect bulb and he gave no room to any further doubts. Failure for an optimist is a chance to start afresh and try a new method. For a pessimist, it is the validation of her fears that she isn't good enough or entitled to success. This is the biggest mindset change you need to make to become an optimist.

Practical Tips

Expect setbacks. You need to know that difficulties and potential setbacks are a part of the game and a necessary prerequisite to toughen you up before success can be achieved.

Stay with your problems for some time. A lot of problems do not have a difficult solution. They just require time and a little patience to wait them out. Stay long with your problems until you are sure they cannot be solved.

Learn from the past. The past is there as a lesson for you. Learn from your previous mistakes and the efforts of other people to avoid the pit-holes they fell into. Do not commit the same mistake twice; once is enough a lesson for you. Repeated mistakes sap away energy and willpower.

CHAPTER TWO

LEARN NOT TO FEAR THE FUTURE

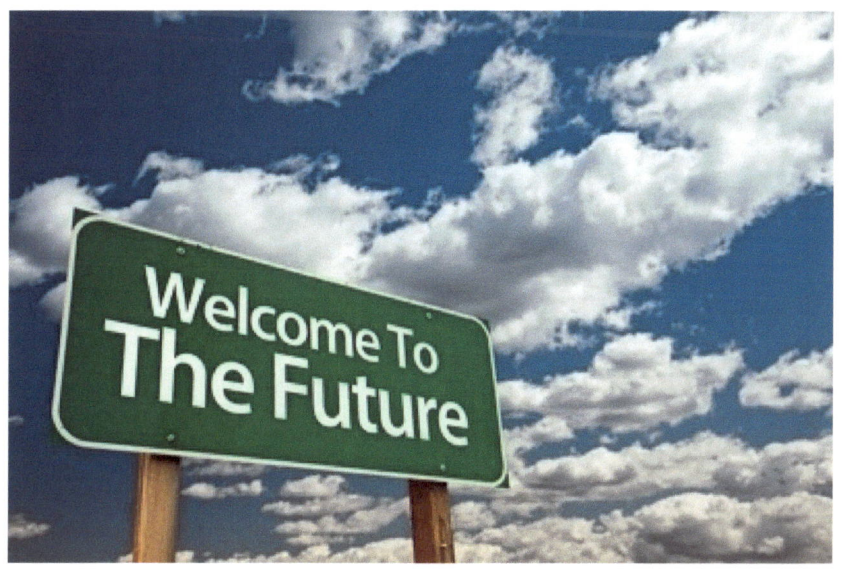

"You realize that our mistrust of the future makes it hard to give up the past."
— Chuck Palahniuk

Our future is not set. There is no such thing as predestination; instead, you write your destiny by the way you think and approach each situation. There is absolutely no reason to fear the future. Your future is only going to become what it is going to be by the way you think and act now. The fear of the unknown has always been a sensitive and paramount emotion in humans from birth. You don't know what tomorrow may bring, so, you are a bit skeptical. Is that normal? Within a certain limit, yes, it is.

There is nothing bad about being cautious or looking well before you leap, just make sure your thoughts do not prevent you from ever making any leaps. Women are more prone to fears. We think it is impossible for things to play out the way we want. Yes, it doesn't always go our way but dreading the future means that at the first setback, you will be ready to turn back. It means that rather than seeing each challenge as an opportunity to learn and become better, you may see them as further proof of your inability to succeed or make a difference. Instead of this, understand that your reactions to the future will determine which future you get to spend; a successful, or regret-filled one.

Practical tips

Do not imagine negative outcomes. If they must occur, then, there is no need to punish you twice. Focusing on them only makes them more liable to occur. Shut them out.

Practice creative visualization and outcomes. Close your eyes for a minute and imagine the action you are about to take successfully. Yes, there are you with your new degree. Yes, that is you in the head office in charge of your department, yes, there you are surrounded by the lovely kids you would like to have while your husband reclines across the room.

Write out the advantages you have. Get a piece of paper and write out what you have going in your favor, your life, health, kids, work, and family. Now, think of how many of them you actively sought to get. If you can get them, what stops you from getting more? Only you!!!

CHAPTER THREE

TRY OUT NEW, UNUSUAL AND DESPERATE THINGS

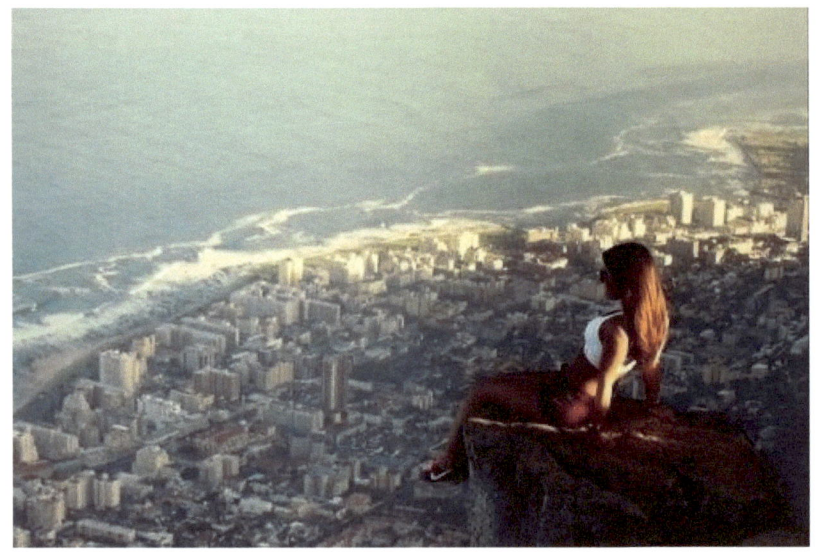

"Only those who will risk going too far can possibly find out how far someone can go."
-T. S. Elliot

    A pessimist only tries out what has been tested and trusted. She doesn't want challenges or to learn new things. She is scared she may not be able to cope with a new routine. She sticks to the usual routine and continues churning out the same generic result every other individual is churning out. To be extraordinary, you need to do extraordinary things, and every new action you try is extraordinary. However, if you have plans of doing great things, then, you need a separate plan far from routine. Do not be scared of new challenges. Believe you can do them. Go unconventional, try out a new system.

Practical Tips

Take action. Another hallmark of pessimism is a reluctance to take on tasks. Pessimists are so sure something will go wrong that they would rather not do anything. You can't be like that. Take on tasks; do not procrastinate or be afraid of getting stressed. As Pablo Picasso said; "Action is the fundamental key to all success."

Try the unusual. Check out a new recipe or a DIY chart for cleaning up your kitchen. A new challenge produces great hormones and sensations that can help you succeed faster.

Chart new paths. Are you in unfamiliar territory? Maybe nobody has ever gotten so far in your particular exploits. Or nobody has ever attempted it. Remember, every road was once just bush. Every action was once just an idea. Your idea can be the next road.

CHAPTER FOUR

BE FLEXIBLE, AMENABLE AND OPEN TO CHANGE

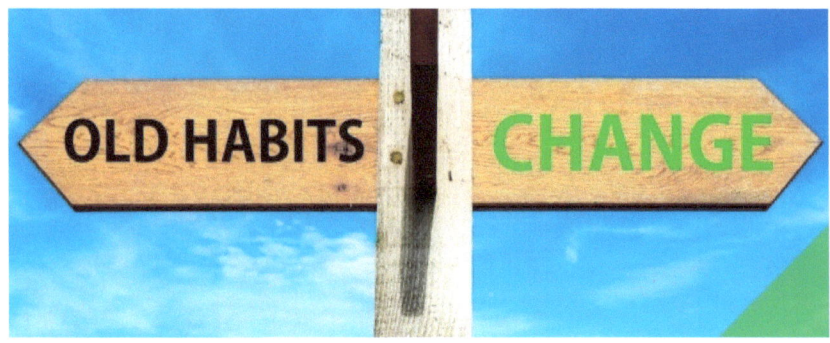

"Don't let goal setting become heavyweights. Remain flexible and allow room for intuitive changes." ― Kelly Martin

A pessimist thrives off already laid plans that guarantee safety and seem to promise minimal risk. Therefore, once she has laid the plans for her that seems to guarantee such a safety net, she becomes unwilling or unable to change them. She cannot bring herself to adjust the plans or modify them for fear of distorting the danger margins she has determined. Her mind binds her from reacting to changes in circumstances. If she does ever try to react, it is only to shift further into negativity. It is often to tell her why she may not succeed.

The thought eats further into her mind, and a vicious cycle develops very quickly robbing her of her decision-making faculty. This means she is less likely to take action and in the improbable case that she does, her pessimism bogs her down and drives her to take evasive or cowardly action. For instance, what would you if you have saved some money towards a new car and then, out of the blues, a promising and bright business idea or opportunity arises? How would a pessimist react?

In most likelihood, she will assuage herself with the reasons why the business may succeed, how she wants a new car and a thousand and one other excuses that will enable her to convince herself not to try a new idea. It will not even matter if she has one or two cars already. It is just the pessimist in her that determines.

Practical Tips

Keep alternatives open. Do not choose a course of action and then immediately turn it into your brain that you will not consider any other line of action no matter the context and subplots that arise. Keep your options as options. Do not close them off.

Draw contingency plans. Learn from the most successful businessmen of all time. Always have a Plan B. This is a bit dicey though. Your plan B does not need always to mean reverting to safety and safe ground. It could be as aggressive as your first plan. It is simply another approach to the issue at hand.

Be fast and smart in reacting. Do not wait till a change is inevitable. The moment you realize that change is prudent, make it. Do not wait till it remains the only option you have.

CHAPTER FIVE

BE POSITIVE

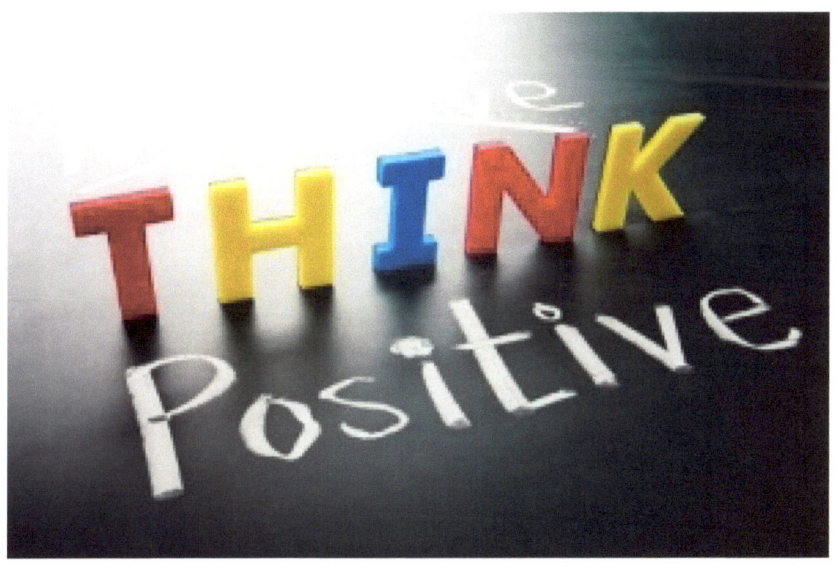

"We can complain because rose bushes have thorns, or rejoice because thorns have roses."
— Alphonse Karr

The quote above aptly sums up the difference between pessimism and optimism. The difference in perspective between an optimist and a pessimist is the key difference between them. This difference though arises from the differing levels of positivity they possess. Do you always seem to be able to find the silver linings in the cloud? Or are you perpetually under a cloud of your troubles? Maybe you even suspect your reactions to your problems are part of the problems too. Welcome to the pessimism club.

By giving in to negative thoughts and assumptions, you leave yourself open to further negative emotions and traits like procrastination, a lack of motivation and a loss of willpower. Allowing negative self-criticism kills off confidence faster than any other thing. Do not give into self-destruction. As Maxwell Maltz said; "Low self-esteem is like driving through life with your handbrake on". Disengage your brakes and free yourself to make meaningful progress.

Practical Tips

Kill the little voice in your head. You know the little voice we talked about before; that one in your head telling you "You can't", "you shouldn't", "It won't", and "It will fail". You need to kill it now. It is hard to succeed already without a voice telling you off right in your brain.

Get motivated. Read up on past successes and people who made it. Get acquainted with their methods and how they achieved a breakthrough. It will keep you motivated and steadfast.

See the opportunity. It is often repeated that opportunities come but once but this is not true.

Opportunities come multiple times. The only catch is that it never comes naked. It is always disguised or hidden under a challenge. Learn to see through and extract opportunities others do not even know it exist.

CHAPTER SIX

PERSEVERANCE; EMPLOY HIBERNATION AND STANDBY MODE TO BEAT HARD TIMES

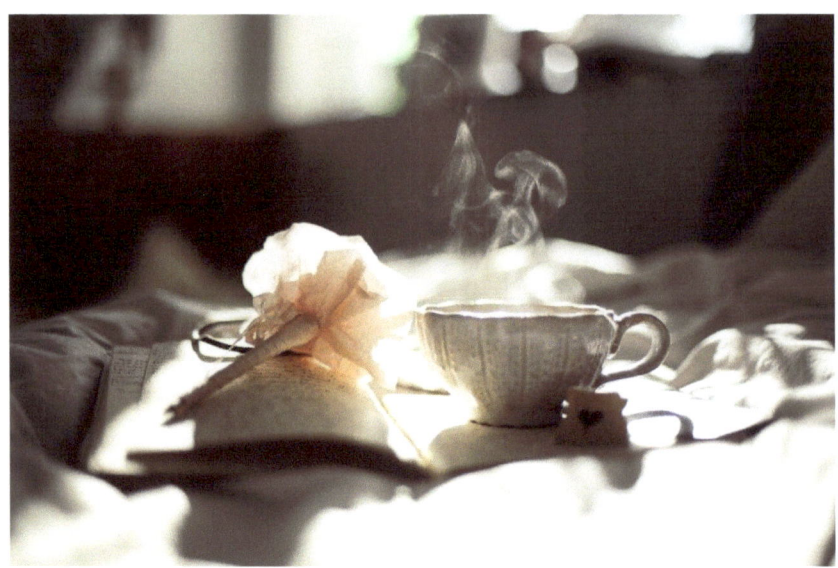

"A hibernating snail does not necessarily mean it is dead."
— Messaoud Mohammed

There is no denying the fact that tough times are going to come and they are definitely going to try your optimism. Even the most optimistic individuals can go down under stress at times. Therefore, you need to prepare ahead for testing times. At times though, one of the biggest problems people have is trying to fight their way through. You can't battle a storm; you can only wrap yourself up against it and wait it out.

When you have realized that this particular storm may be inevitable or a bit too heavy for you to fight, do not expend precious energy on a wasted cause. Instead, batten down your tents and prepare to hibernate until it passes. Maybe a spouse or partner is going through a lot of work-related stress and can't seem to give you enough time. Do not attempt to fight him on it. Time cannot heal everything, but patience can heal every wound. In the words of Fulton J. Sheen; "Patience is not an absence of action, rather it is "timing". It waits for the right time to act, for the right principles and in the right way." Be wise enough to know when you need to exercise patience.

Practical Tips

Understand your problem. Understanding your problem is definitely non-negotiable. Do not stumble around in the dark. Identify and gauge what you are up against. That will tell you whether you need the flight or fight response.

Prepare while waiting. Do not be like the snail that just hibernates. Make hay while you wait. Learn new skills and prepare yourself ahead of the action. Add more value and abilities while you wait out the storm.

Plan your route. While you wait, there is ample time to draw up a plan of action. Utilize that time to judicious effect by taking the chance to create a plan under little pressure.

CHAPTER SEVEN

DO NOT GET ISOLATED; DECIDE, COMMUNICATE, INTERACT AND BE IN THE THICK OF ACTION.

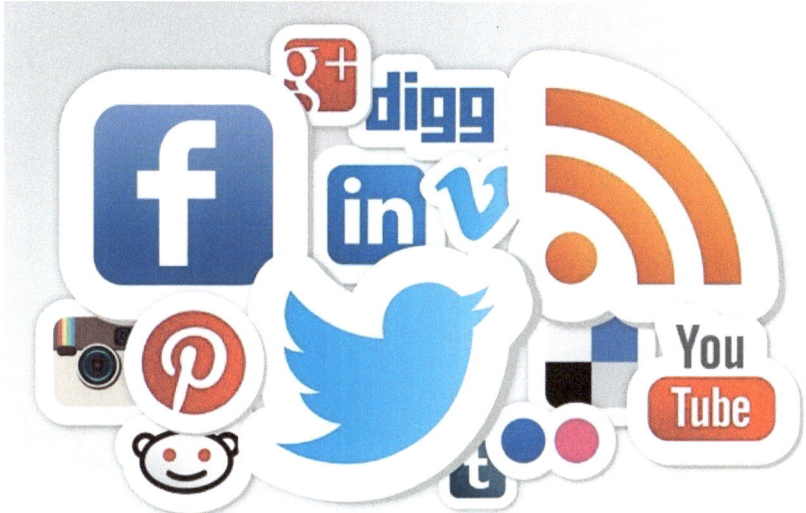

"Take responsibility for your happiness; never put it in other people's hands."
― *Roy T. Bennett*

One way to remain in control of your success, happiness, and destiny is by ensuring that it never gets out of your own hands. Do not take perseverance to mean endless waiting or a call to remain inactive. Instead, take control of your actions and make your destiny. Do not allow the outcome of your action or efforts to remain too dependent on what other people do or think of you. Remain in the thick of the action, understand what is going on at each step and be positively involved. Do not leave your marriage or work to your partner or colleagues to create a direction all on their own. Chances are you may not like their direction or spin.

Take absolute control and be involved in making the decisions you follow. Do not wait for others to map out a strategy for you to follow. Utilize the people around you, derive support and extract teamwork from them, but do not make yourself ignorant.

Practical tips

Provide clear communication. Be wary of sending false signals. Do not make the mistake of throwing false signals to people. Be clear, concise, and detailed in communication.

Build a network of support. The people around you are a great source of motivation when you are down. Tap into the positive encouragement and the support they offer your efforts.

Help the people around you. As humans, ideally, we are pleased when we can help less-privileged people around us. No matter how bad your situation is, there is always somebody in the next room feeling worse. Reach out to them, help them and encourage them. Give out love; identify and support somebody weaker than you.

CHAPTER EIGHT

BE GRATEFUL FOR WHAT YOU HAVE

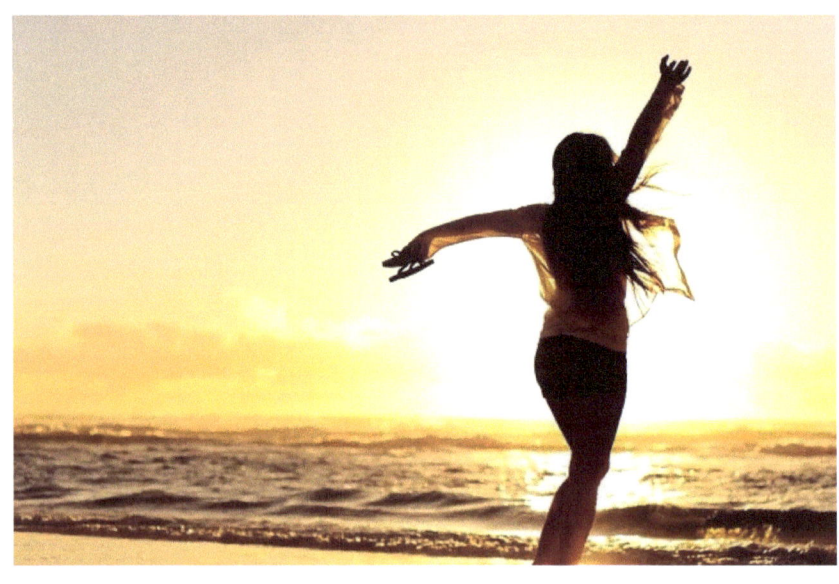

"Be grateful for what you already have while you pursue your goals. If you aren't grateful for what you already have, what makes you think you would be happy with more."
— Roy T. Bennett

Gratitude for what you have been able to achieve helps optimism in a way few things can. It is motivation for your optimism. No matter how little, our body reacts positively when we can recount the progress we have made. This makes us more likely to be able to see positives. It gives us the belief that if we could have made such progress, then, we can create even further milestones. An ungrateful mind is a negative mind. Being unable to see your progress and achievement will leave you in reverse mode.

When we are grateful, we are happy, and when we are happy, we are more likely to stick to what we are doing for longer. Be happy for what others have done to you. It will make them interested in doing more. Be happy for the extra edge you have, the things in your favor and the things you have done.

Practical Tips

Be happy with the small steps. Some successes arrive as sudden breakthroughs, but they are very rare. Invest in the power of small steps and use them to build your way up the ladder. Each progress is positive, small or big. Just don't stay stagnant.

List your achievements. Anytime you feel downcast, create time and pick out a sheet of paper. List out the times you succeeded against all odds. Lean back in your chair and practice the opposite of creative visualization. Think back to your previous success. Drink in the memory of success and refuel your engine for a long-haul once again.

Reward yourself. Give yourself small treats when you complete milestones and make progress. Buy yourself a favorite meal, take in a new movie or spend some quality time alone at a spa or beach. Just make yourself happy that you did the little you did. It could be essential.

CHAPTER NINE

CREATE A BUFFER-ZONE

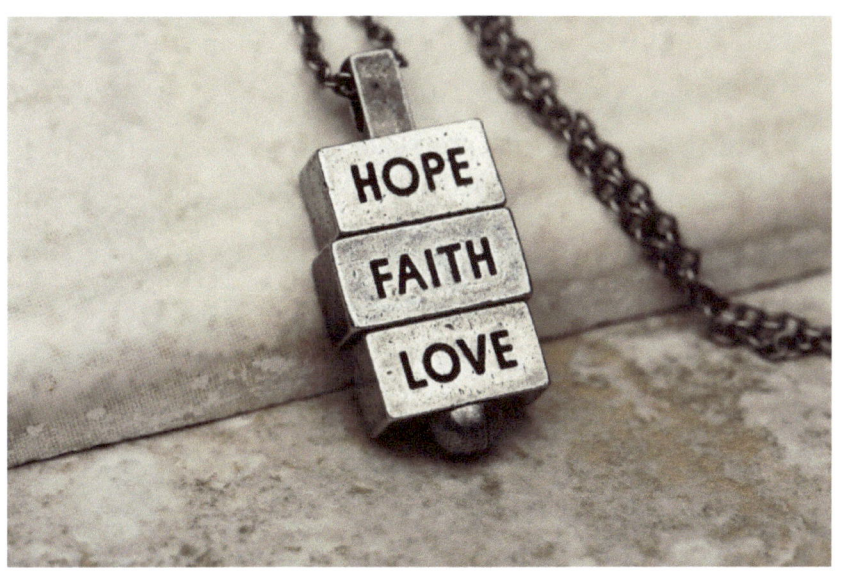

"There's no harm in hoping for the best as long as you're prepared for the worst."
— Stephen King

Pessimism may be very wrong, but discretion remains a great part of valor. Sadly, there is such a thing as being too optimistic. Optimism does not ask that you lose your eyes, it only asks for undivided loyalty and hope from deep within your mind. The line between plain foolhardiness and optimism can be quite thin. It can be a bit hard to judge where optimism stops being that and becomes baseless stubbornness and obduracy. As much as pessimism has hampered many people, an equally sizable number of people have lost out by chasing lost causes.

Therefore, learning the right causes to devote and dedicate your optimism too, is an integral part of building the optimism in the first place. Not all endeavors, relationships or efforts are meant to be successful. We may not know which ones are doomed to fail before starting, but you should not hesitate to pull out of any exertion that seems to promise the only failure.

Practical Tips

Listen to the alarms. It can be tough to separate the two initially, but your intuition is different from the little voice at the back of your head. Your intuition is an alarm bell wired permanently into your prefrontal cortex to supply you with genuine warnings. Listen to it when it sounds; it is almost always right.

It is never too late to pull out. The only thing worse than doing the wrong thing is remaining stuck doing the wrong things. It is never too late to pull out of a fruitless pursuit. Save yourself the extra stress and preserve as much optimism as you can.

Do not be guided by sentiments. I know we make our decisions based on sentiments. I know they determine a lot of our actions, but you cannot allow your optimism to blind you to the realities on the ground. Do not allow love to stop you from seeing the flaws of your partner. Instead, work with him to correct it. Probe your optimism. Is it based on cold, hard logic, calculations and intuition, or simply driven by sentiments?

CONCLUSION

Why should you become an optimist?

Why do I want you always to keep your hopes high even in the face of stark prospects? Why should you abandon the "safety-first" mode of thinking? If you have read this book, I know you must have the answers, but let me help you recapture the essence of optimism.

Optimism is being able to look at any situation or embark or any pursuits with genuinely sincere hopes of succeeding. It is standing firm under the assumption that you are capable and entitled to success and happiness as much as anybody. Optimism protects you from getting browbeaten by difficult situations even when you are disadvantaged. It is the one trait the greatest personalities and leaders from Jesus, Cleopatra, Mohammed down to Rev Martin Luther King, and Nelson Mandela possessed in spades. All these people were able to keep going down the tunnel in the firm believed that there was a light at the end.

Optimism needs to be a part of you. As a woman, you have even more reasons to pay attention to the balance between the positivity and negativity within you. The mother is the primary determinant of a family's mood and demeanor. You control the pulse and temperature of relationships, and you are more prone to the ill effects of pessimism. Therefore, it is not a choice for you to keep breeding negativity within your mind. You cannot allow your mind to get overgrown by the weeds of pessimism.

However, even though optimism means to keep going down the tunnel in firm belief, knowing for certain that there is a tunnel, and is the first substrate of optimism. Do not plan to scratch out a tunnel from the bare rock with your hands. Be sure the tunnel is there first and not flooded. Do not be afraid to turn back and try another tunnel if you find a block ahead in your tunnel. The central tenet of optimism is to keep your foot firmly and decisively on the accelerator, hardly yielding and continuously moving. It doesn't matter if the progress is slow. The most important thing is that your leg is down on the accelerator, ready to ease up on the gas when you need to wait or change gears. Do not forget how to step on the brakes though, when it becomes necessary. You need both pedals to drive your car to success and happiness.

Why should you not be a pessimist?

Why should you squash that little voice trying to dominate you and keep you dry and above tide? Why should you learn when to apply the brakes and not keep the pedal down at all time?

Well, pessimism has to be the most illogical mode of thinking. Pessimism teaches you to fear failure; then, tells you not to try hard because you can't fail if you don't try. Take a moment to digest that. Pessimism conveniently fails to inform you that you can't succeed without trying too. The worst single fact about pessimists is that they fear both failure and success. They are afraid to fail and afraid of succeeding. They feel an initial success may be unsustainable. Therefore, they don't try to succeed initially. They simply keep trying to be safe. What they forget is that life has no guarantees. Trying to be safe does not mean you will remain secure.

I will rather take my chances, open my wings and fly high in the hope that I may succeed rather than remain on the ground, wings folded, eyes downcast and choose not to consider my chances in the vain hope that life might leave me alone and safe. I will rather not be left alone. I will rather move than sit down permanently. I will rather write my tomorrow than wake up tomorrow. I will rather cast my destiny and mold it than wait for the one that life decides to throw at me. I will rather hunt for food than remain huddled praying that I don't get hunted. I will rather hope than sulk. I will rather try than hide. I will rather lift off and fly high than chase safety on the ground. Wouldn't you?

I leave you with these wise words of the great Indian statesman, Mahatma Gandhi that I have pasted underneath my mirror. Maybe you should too. He said;

"Man often becomes what he believes himself to be. If I keep on saying to myself that I cannot do a certain thing, it is possible that I may end up by really becoming incapable of doing it. On the contrary, if I have the belief that I can do it, I shall surely acquire the capacity to do it even if I may not have it at the beginning."

I want to thank you and congratulate you for buying this book!

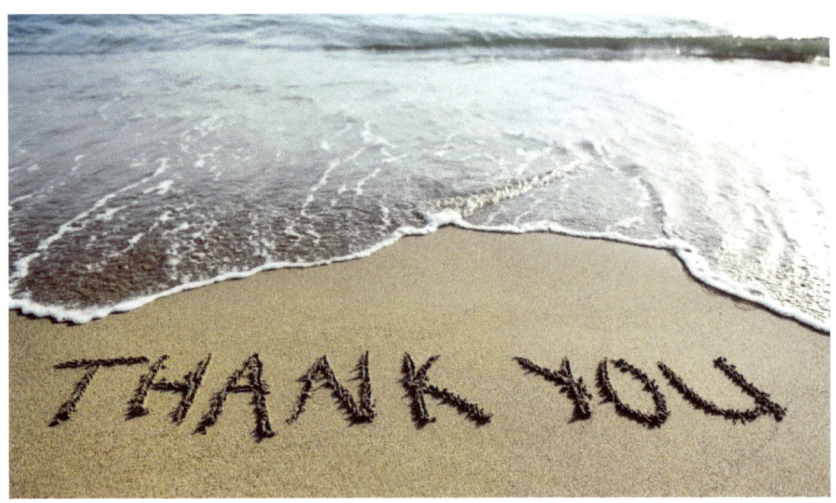

www.ingramcontent.com/pod-product-compliance
Lightning Source LLC
Chambersburg PA
CBHW041942240526
45473CB00033B/428